TUBAL LIGATION RECOVERY DIET

A Comprehensive Guide To Nutritional Support, Female Sterilization And Fallopian Tube Recovery

DR LUCAS KAYCE

DISCLAIMER

This book about illness and nutrition is not meant to replace expert medical advice, diagnosis, or treatment; rather, it is meant purely for informational reasons. This book's content is founded on broad concepts and recommendations for managing diseases and nutrition.

Before adopting any major dietary or lifestyle changes, readers are recommended to speak with a qualified healthcare provider, such as a licensed physician or registered dietitian, especially if they have pre-existing medical concerns. Everybody has different health demands, so what works for one person might not work for another.

The use of the information provided in this book may have unfavorable repercussions or consequences, for which the author and publisher disclaim all liability. No disease is meant to be identified, treated, cured, or prevented by the information provided.

The book may include contain references to medical literature or research findings; however readers are urged to independently confirm this material and contact reliable sources.

It is important to remember that the fields of nutrition and medicine are always changing, and that new findings could have an impact on the advice offered in this book. As a result, readers are urged to keep up with the most recent advancements in healthcare and, when in doubt, seek professional counsel.

By reading this book, readers agree that they are in charge of their own health decisions and release the author and publisher from any liability arising from the use of the material in the book, whether direct or indirect.

TABLE OF CONTENTS

ABOUT THE BOOK

The book, "Tubal Ligation Recovery Diet," tackles a critical component of women's health by giving thorough guidance to diet throughout the post-tubal ligation recovery period. In the introduction section, the backdrop of tubal ligation is reviewed, underlining the goal of the book and how the proposed recovery diet assists the healing process.

The book digs into understanding tubal ligation, covering the numerous ways and typical reasons for undergoing this treatment. The chapter also provides an overview of the recovery period, setting the stage for the need for a well-planned recovery diet.

The book highlights the significance of nutrition in the recovery process, emphasizing the role of a balanced diet in post-surgery healing. It investigates how diet directly affects healing and enumerates the benefits of adhering to a carefully selected recovery diet.

It educates readers on building a foundation for recovery, highlighting the necessity of consulting with healthcare specialists, preparing psychologically and emotionally, and establishing realistic expectations for the recovery process.

It also includes practical guidance on dietary requirements for tubal ligation recovery, emphasizing on nutrient-rich meals important for healing. Specific focus is paid to proteins, vitamins, minerals, water, fiber, and healthy fats.

The book walks readers through the process of meal planning for recovery, providing insight into constructing balanced meals and providing sample meal plans for breakfast, lunch, supper, and snacks, along with hydration advice.

It tackles common concerns and obstacles during recovery, such as nausea, digestive issues, weight control, and food aversions, while addressing unique dietary limitations.

It emphasizes the necessity of mild exercise during recuperation, addressing the types of recommended activities and outlining a gradual return to physical activity.

It also focuses on emotional well-being during recovery, recognizing challenges, and providing coping skills, along with the significance of seeking help.

The book focuses beyond the immediate healing phase, examining long-term dietary considerations, post-recovery nutrition, maintaining a healthy lifestyle, and the significance of follow-up with healthcare providers.

Overall, this book serves as a helpful resource for persons following tubal ligation, offering practical advice on the essential role diet plays in the recovery process and providing a path for a balanced and healthy post-surgical journey.

TUBAL LIGATION RECOVERY DIET OVERVIEW

BACKGROUND OF TUBAL LIGATION

Tubal ligation, generally known as "getting one's tubes tied," is a surgical treatment meant for permanent contraception in women. This elective treatment involves the blocking, sealing, or cutting of the fallopian tubes, stopping the eggs from migrating from the ovaries to the uterus. By stopping this important pathway, tubal ligation successfully ensures that sperm cannot reach the egg, thereby preventing fertilization.

Historically, tubal ligation has been a widely chosen technique of contraception for women seeking a permanent answer to family planning. The roots of this operation can be traced back to the mid-20th century when surgical procedures were perfected and safety requirements increased. Initially, it gained popularity as a technique for reducing family size, and over the years, its scope has evolved to incorporate medical and personal issues.

The treatment is generally deemed safe and effective, but individuals need to grasp the permanence of the decision and thoroughly analyze its repercussions before proceeding.

Despite its widespread use, tubal ligation has not been without controversy. Debates have revolved around problems of autonomy, informed consent, and the age at which individuals should be permitted to have treatment. Additionally, developments in contraceptive technologies have led to discussions about other, less invasive choices. Understanding the historical backdrop and developing viewpoints surrounding tubal ligation is vital for those contemplating this choice, as it entails not only medical surgery but also a very personal decision with long-term ramifications.

HOW THE RECOVERY DIET SUPPORTS HEALING

The postoperative time following tubal ligation is a vital step in a woman's road toward recovery. During this time, the body undergoes healing and rebuilding, and a good diet plays a vital part in aiding this process. The recovery diet is particularly intended to deliver critical nutrients, enhance tissue healing, and limit potential problems.

An important component of the recovery diet is providing an adequate amount of protein. Protein is vital for the creation of new tissues and the healing of cells injured after surgery.

Incorporating lean sources of protein, such as poultry, fish, tofu, and beans, helps boost the body's healing capacity. Moreover, a balanced diet rich in vitamins and minerals, notably vitamin C and zinc, stimulates the immune system and improves wound healing.

Hydration is another key part of the recovery diet. Staying well-hydrated aids in the clearance of toxins from the body and helps maintain proper organ function. Adequate fluid consumption also avoids dehydration, a major worry post-surgery, and contributes to the overall well-being of the individual.

In addition to specific nutrients, the recovery diet emphasizes the significance of a well-balanced and readily digestible meal plan. Foods that are soft on the digestive tract, such as fruits, vegetables, whole grains, and lean proteins, are encouraged. These choices promote regular bowel movements, lower the risk of constipation, and help general comfort during the recovery period.

It is vital to remember that individual nutritional demands may vary, and consultation with a healthcare expert or a qualified dietitian is advisable to adjust the recovery diet to unique conditions. By embracing a nutritionally sound approach during the recovery phase, individuals can maximize their healing process and enhance their general well-being after undergoing tubal ligation.

CHAPTER ONE

UNDERSTANDING TUBAL LIGATION

WHAT IS TUBAL LIGATION?

Tubal ligation, frequently referred to as "getting one's tubes tied," is a surgical treatment aimed to permanently prevent conception by closing or sealing the fallopian tubes. The fallopian tubes are key components of the female reproductive system, functioning as channels for eggs to migrate from the ovaries to the uterus. When these tubes are clogged, the eggs are unable to meet with sperm, essentially blocking fertilization. This technique of contraception is considered a permanent form of birth control, and its effectiveness is high, with a low failure rate.

COMMON REASONS FOR TUBAL LIGATION

Various causes drive individuals to decide on tubal ligation. One prevalent motivation is the desire for a long-term or permanent answer to family planning. Some individuals may choose tubal ligation because they have reached a point in their lives when they are certain they do not want to have more children. This decision can be influenced by factors such as age, financial stability, and personal or medical considerations. Tubal ligation is also selected by persons who want to avoid potential adverse effects or hormonal changes connected with other forms of birth control.

DIFFERENT METHODS OF TUBAL LIGATION

There are numerous strategies performed in tubal ligation procedures. One frequent procedure is laparoscopic tubal ligation, when small incisions are made in the belly, and a tiny camera and equipment are used to access and close up the fallopian tubes. Another procedure is mini-laparotomy, involving a wider incision commonly performed in the lower abdomen. During this surgery, the fallopian tubes are reached directly for closure. Additionally, there is the possibility of hysteroscopic tubal ligation, which entails blocking the tubes through the cervix with the assistance of a hysteroscope.

The patient's health, medical history, and the surgeon's experience all play a role in the method selection.

OVERVIEW OF THE RECUPERATION PERIOD

After having a tubal ligation, patients may anticipate a time of recuperation during which they should follow certain guidelines and may feel some discomfort. Despite being less invasive, laparoscopic tubal ligation still requires abdominal surgery, and recovery time may be several days. In the area of the incisions, pain, swelling, and bruising are typical, although they usually go away in a week or two. To encourage healing, physical activity, and heavy lifting should be minimized during the first phase of recuperation. To guarantee a speedy recovery and lower the chance of complications, patients must adhere to the post-operative care guidelines given by their healthcare experts.

Tubal ligation, which includes blocking or closing the fallopian tubes, is a permanent method of birth control. A person's decision to have this surgery done is frequently impacted by personal, health, or family planning factors. Various techniques, such as hysteroscopic tubal ligation, mini-laparotomy, and laparoscopic tubal ligation, provide possibilities customized to meet specific needs. While recovery from tubal ligation varies, it usually entails some discomfort and a reduced activity level to promote healing. It is crucial that anyone thinking about tubal ligation carefully considers their alternatives with medical professionals and balances the permanence of this procedure against their desired number of children.

CHAPTER TWO

THE ROLE OF NUTRITION IN HEALING

NUTRITION'S FUNCTION IN POST-SURGERY RECOVERY

The body's capacity to heal after surgery depends in large part on nutrition, which affects the body's capacity to fight infections, restore damaged tissues, and regain strength. The body experiences increased stress following surgery, necessitating the need for more nutrients to aid in the healing process. Sufficient nourishment is vital for wound healing because it supplies the building blocks needed for the synthesis of new tissue and the restoration of damaged cells. Specifically, protein plays a key role in the production of collagen, a protein necessary for tissue regeneration and wound closure.

Vitamins and minerals are essential in the post-surgery phase, in addition to protein. Zinc is necessary for cell division and tissue healing, while vitamin C is necessary for collagen formation and immune system function.

These micronutrients participate in several metabolic reactions that are essential to the cascade of healing. Therefore, to support the body's increased nutritional requirements throughout the recuperation phase, a diet rich in nutrients and well-balanced is essential.

HOW NUTRITION IMPACTS THE HEALING PROCESS

Dietary practices have a significant effect on the healing process, affecting both the physiological and psychological components of rehabilitation. Eating well can reduce the chance of problems and shorten the time needed for recuperation. An immune system that is weak or unbalanced may increase the body's susceptibility to infections and impede the healing process.

In addition, inadequate nourishment may result in wasting muscles, low energy, and general weakness, which will make it more difficult for the patient to recover from surgery and become functional again.

It's important to consider how diet affects recuperation psychologically in addition as physiologically. Mood, mental clarity, and general well-being can all be positively impacted by a well-planned and nutrient-rich diet. On the other hand, an inadequate diet could exacerbate emotions of exhaustion, agitation, and tension, impeding the psychological part of healing. Thus, in addition to providing for the body's dietary needs, medical practitioners stress the significance of treating patients' emotional and mental health as part of a comprehensive post-surgery care plan.

ADVANTAGES OF A WELL-DESIGNED RECUPERATION DIET

There are several advantages to a carefully thought-out healing diet that go far beyond the first few weeks following surgery. The development of ideal wound healing and tissue restoration is one of the main benefits. Protein, vitamins, and minerals are among the nutrients that help create new blood vessels and promote collagen synthesis and tissue regeneration.

Consequently, this reduces the likelihood of scarring and improves the general healing process.

In addition, a recovery diet rich in nutrients helps avoid issues like inflammation and infections. Sufficient nourishment is essential for the immune system to work well, and a healthy body is better able to fight off any enemies. This lowers the possibility of surgical site infections while enhancing the body's capacity to control inflammation, which is essential to the healing process.

A proper recovery diet is essential for preserving or gaining back strength and muscle mass in addition to the physical components. In particular, protein is necessary for the synthesis of muscle protein, which helps to prevent muscular atrophy and weakening during the recuperation phase. For patients hoping to recover their mobility and functionality after surgery, this is crucial.

CHAPTER THREE

LAYING THE GROUNDWORK FOR HEALING

SPEAKING WITH MEDICAL EXPERTS

Creating a foundation for rehabilitation requires a multidimensional strategy that takes mental, emotional, and physical health into account. Consulting with medical experts is an important part of this procedure. Consulting with medical professionals guarantees a thorough comprehension of the ailment, the range of treatment alternatives, and individualized advice catered to the unique requirements of each patient. By offering knowledge, assistance, and continual progress monitoring, healthcare providers are essential in building a strong basis for rehabilitation.

GETTING READY EMOTIONALLY AND MENTALLY

In the healing process, mental and emotional preparation are just as important. It can be emotionally draining to confront a health issue, and long-term treatment success requires attending to the mental parts of the process. This includes learning to be resilient, having an optimistic outlook, and creating coping techniques to get through the emotional ups and downs that frequently accompany a health crisis. Individual or group therapy can offer helpful strategies for handling stress, anxiety, and other emotional difficulties, building a solid basis for the healing process.

RECOVERING WITH REASONABLE EXPECTATIONS

One of the most important things that can help people navigate their route to wellness with a balanced perspective is setting reasonable expectations for recovery. Setting unrealistic expectations might impede progress by causing irritation and disappointment. Support networks and medical professionals are essential in helping people set realistic objectives and benchmarks. Understanding that healing is a progressive process with ups and downs makes for a more positive and long-lasting strategy. People can enjoy little achievements, stay motivated, and remain dedicated to their recovery process by having reasonable expectations.

Laying the groundwork for recovery necessitates a team effort that includes talking with medical experts, getting ready psychologically and emotionally, and having reasonable expectations. Every one of these ideas contributes differently to helping people on their journey to well-being and guarantees a thorough and all-encompassing approach to healing. People can create the foundation for a fruitful and long-lasting recovery path by working well with healthcare professionals, developing mental and emotional fortitude, and adopting reasonable expectations.

CHAPTER FOUR

NUTRITIONAL RECOMMENDATIONS FOR TUBAL LIGATION HEALING

SYNOPSIS OF THE RECUPERATION DIET

Focusing on a nutritious and well-balanced recovery diet is essential following tubal ligation, a surgical surgery that blocks the fallopian tubes to permanently prevent conception. During the healing process, a healthy diet can be very helpful in fostering healing, lowering inflammation, and maintaining general health at its best. A range of nutrient-dense meals that assist the body's healing processes and supply vital vitamins and minerals should be included in the recovery diet.

FOODS HIGH IN NUTRIENTS FOR HEALING

Including foods that are high in nutrients and provide an abundance of vitamins, minerals, and antioxidants is a crucial component of the recovery diet. These meals help the body heal wounds, strengthen the immune system, and lower the chance of problems.

Fruits and vegetables, whole grains, lean meats, dairy products, and dairy substitutes are a few examples of these foods. Making sure the dish is vibrant and varied will contribute to providing a wide range of nutrients required for a quick and efficient recovery.

PROTEINS

As the basic building blocks of all tissues, proteins are essential to the healing process that occurs after tubal ligation. It's crucial to include lean protein sources including fish, poultry, lean meats, eggs, dairy products, and plant-based protein options like tofu and beans. Consuming enough protein promotes immune system function, decreases muscle loss, and supports tissue repair—all of which contribute to a speedier recovery.

MINERALS AND VITAMINS

The consumption of vitamins and minerals is a key component of a well-rounded recovery diet as they are essential for the healing process. Citrus fruits and vegetables include vitamin C, which aids in the creation of collagen and the healing of wounds. Nuts, seeds, and whole grains are good sources of zinc, which is essential for tissue healing and immune system performance. Including vitamin-rich leafy greens, vibrant veggies, and whole grains also offers a wide variety of nutrients required for the best possible recuperation.

DRINKING PLENTY OF WATER

Although it is frequently disregarded, maintaining adequate hydration is essential for healing following any surgical treatment, including tubal ligation. Maintaining adequate hydration promotes healthy biological functioning, facilitates the removal of toxins, and helps avoid constipation, which is a common issue during the healing process. To make sure you're getting enough water, clear broths, and herbal teas are great options.

FIBER

Consuming dietary fiber is crucial for preserving gut health, particularly after surgery when reduced mobility may occur. Consuming a diet high in fruits, vegetables, whole grains, and legumes can help reduce constipation, which is a typical side effect of painkillers and surgery. Moreover, fiber promotes a balanced gut microbiota, which enhances general well-being when recovering.

GOOD FATS

A recovery diet that includes healthy fats is crucial for several body processes, including as hormone generation and fat-soluble vitamin absorption. Olive oil, almonds, seeds, avocados, and fatty fish are good sources of healthful fats. These fats support a feeling of fullness in addition to offering vital nutrients, assisting people in keeping a healthy, well-balanced diet while they heal.

After tubal ligation, a well-thought-out recuperation diet ought to emphasize meals high in nutrients, such as enough protein, vitamins, minerals, water, fiber, and healthy fats.

CHAPTER FIVE

ORGANIZING YOUR MEALS TO RECOVER

MAKING WELL-COMPOSED MEALS

Whether recuperating from an illness, surgery, or intense physical exercise, balanced meals are essential. These meals should contain a variety of vitamins and minerals in addition to a well-balanced combination of macronutrients such as proteins, carbs, and healthy fats. The objective is to give the body the vital nutrients it needs for the best possible healing and regeneration.

The unique dietary needs of each person must be taken into account while preparing balanced meals for recuperation. For instance, a person recovering from surgery could need more protein to help with tissue regeneration, whereas a person recovering from a protracted illness might need a balance of carbs for energy and nutrients that support the immune system. Getting advice from a nutritionist or medical expert might help you customize meals to fit your needs.

EXAMPLE MENUS

During recuperation, sample meal plans can be a useful tool for attaining a balanced diet. These programs must be adaptable, taking nutritional requirements and individual preferences into account. A normal day could begin with a filling breakfast, be followed by a variety of lunch and dinner selections, and be punctuated with high-nutrient snacks.

FOR BREAKFAST

A breakfast consisting of fruits, lean proteins, and nutritious grains could be geared toward healing. For example, oatmeal with fresh berries and Greek yogurt on top offers a good balance of antioxidants, high-quality protein, and complex carbohydrates.

This helps with the immune system and muscle restoration in addition to providing long-lasting energy for the rest of the day.

LUNCH

Lunch can include a range of vibrant vegetables, healthy fats, and lean proteins. A dish full of mixed vegetables and quinoa topped with grilled chicken or tofu is nutrient-dense. Including a healthy fat source, such as avocado or olive oil, improves the way fat-soluble vitamins are absorbed and increases feelings of fullness all around.

DINNER

Make sure your dinner includes a variety of nutrients. Complex carbs, vital vitamins, and omega-3 fatty acids can all be found in a piece of baked salmon served with steamed broccoli and sweet potatoes. This mixture aids in the reduction of inflammation and promotes general healing.

MUNCHIES

Between-meal snacks present a chance to add extra nutrients. Nut and seed mixtures, sliced veggies with hummus, or Greek yogurt with honey and walnuts can all be filling choices. These snacks supply vital micronutrients and help sustain energy levels over the day.

TIPS FOR HYDRATION

Maintaining sufficient hydration is essential for recuperation since water is essential for multiple physiological functions such as digestion, assimilation of nutrients, and control of body temperature. People going through recovery should try to drink the same amount of water all day long. Flavor-enhancing and hydrating herbal teas, broths, and infused water with fruit or herb slices can be made.

To sum up, meal planning for recovery is all about preparing meals that are nutritionally sound and well-balanced. Individuals can design wholesome and fulfilling breakfasts, lunches, dinners, and snacks with the help of sample meal plans. Sustaining adequate hydration is also crucial for promoting general healing and well-being.

CHAPTER SIX

HANDLING FREQUENTLY ASKED QUESTIONS AND DIFFICULTIES

MANAGING NAUSEA AND DIGESTIVE PROBLEMS

One of the most difficult parts of the healing process can be navigating the frequently painful landscape of nausea and digestive problems while in recovery. Adopting a mindful eating strategy that emphasizes smaller, more often meals over larger servings may help patients feel better.

Choosing foods that are easy to digest, such as rice, bananas, or plain crackers, can help reduce discomfort. Furthermore, it's critical to maintain water because dehydration can make stomach issues worse.

Try brewing different herbal teas and steer clear of oily or spicy foods to help soothe your tummy.

KEEPING A HEALTHY WEIGHT DURING RECOVERY

For people going through recovery, maintaining a healthy weight is crucial. It's critical to strike a balance between giving the body the nourishment it needs to mend itself and avoiding uncontrollably losing or gaining weight. Working together with medical specialists, such as dietitians, can provide tailored advice. A balanced diet can be supported by emphasizing nutrient-dense foods including lean meats, complete grains, and an assortment of fruits and vegetables. A comprehensive approach to weight management during the healing process is ensured by routinely tracking weight variations and modifying meal regimens accordingly.

OVERCOMING FOOD AVERSIONS

It's critical to approach meals with flexibility and inventiveness as food aversions can provide a substantial obstacle to the healing process.

Replacing monotony in the diet with variations in preparation techniques, textures, and flavor profiles can assist. Over time, aversions may be overcome by introducing undesired foods gradually and combining them into cuisines that you already know and love. Support from family members and medical experts can be quite helpful in offering inspiration and encouragement during this difficult journey.

SPECIAL THOUGHTS REGARDING DIETARY LIMITATIONS

When following dietary limitations, people must negotiate a challenging environment to make sure their nutritional requirements are satisfied. It becomes crucial to communicate with nutritionists and healthcare professionals to choose which foods to include and avoid. A balanced diet can be maintained by looking into alternate sources of vital nutrients, such as plant-based proteins or gluten-free cereals. Carefully reading food labels and looking for goods or recipes designed to fit particular dietary requirements can enable people to make educated decisions while following their recommended dietary plans. Those coping with particular dietary issues during recovery may find that participating in continuing education and support groups offers insightful information and encouraging words.

Resolving common issues and difficulties within the framework of recovery necessitates a multidimensional strategy that takes into account each person's requirements, preferences, and medical circumstances. Through customized approaches to address nausea, adjust for weight changes, get over food aversions, and work with dietary constraints, people can make more progress toward recovery and long-term health.

CHAPTER SEVEN

EXERCISE AND PHYSICAL ACTIVITY

THE VALUE OF MODERATE EXERCISE

Exercise and physical activity are essential for preserving general health and well-being. The value of mild exercise is one important factor, especially for people with different degrees of fitness and health issues. Gentle exercise is an inclusive method that can be used by people who are just starting in fitness or who have physical limitations. Low-impact motions that enhance muscular strength, flexibility, and cardiovascular health without placing undue strain on the joints characterize this type of exercise.

Mild exercise has several advantages, such as better mood, higher energy, and better circulation. It is especially helpful for people managing chronic diseases or recuperating from injuries. Walking, swimming, and yoga are just a few examples of the many activities that are considered gentle exercises.

These activities offer a fun and sustainable approach to adding physical activity to everyday life, and they can be customized to match the needs of each individual.

EXERCISE TYPES THAT ARE SUGGESTED

When it comes to suggested workout regimens, a wide variety of activities make up a thorough fitness regimen. Exercises that increase heart health and endurance include swimming, cycling, and jogging.

Muscle tone and bone density are improved by strength training, which includes workouts using your body weight or weightlifting. Stretching and yoga are examples of flexibility activities that increase joint mobility and lower the risk of injury.

Exercise routine variety not only keeps things interesting but also addresses various facets of physical fitness. Combining aerobic, strength, and flexibility training improves general health and fosters a well-rounded, long-lasting fitness program. People are motivated and made to feel good about them when they select activities that suit their interests and fitness objectives.

PROGRESSIVE RESUMPTION OF EXERCISE

A gradual return to physical exercise is necessary following a period of idleness or when recovering from a disease or accident. Hurrying into strenuous exercise might cause injuries and impede one's progress. A gradual approach lowers the chance of setbacks by allowing the body to adjust to higher activity levels. People may begin with low-impact workouts at first, working their way up to more demanding ones as their fitness level increases.

Seeking advice from fitness specialists or medical professionals can offer tailored recommendations for a safe transition back to physical activity.

During this shift, listening to one's body and setting reasonable goals are essential. Gradual increases in both length and intensity, along with appropriate warm-up and cool-down protocols, help to promote a more seamless transition back into regular exercise. By reducing the chance of injury and promoting enjoyment, this method paves the way for a long-lasting and sustainable commitment to physical well-being.

CHAPTER EIGHT

EMOTIONAL HEALTH THROUGHOUT REHAB

IDENTIFYING EMOTIONAL DIFFICULTIES

Identifying and accepting emotional difficulties is a critical first step on the road to recovery and general well-being. Emotional difficulties can take many different forms, from irritation and rage to worry and sadness. Being aware of these emotional cues is crucial for those in recovery because they frequently have a big impact on the healing process as a whole. Being able to recognize particular triggers and comprehend the underlying reasons for emotional difficulties can enable people to take proactive measures to resolve these problems.

The dread of relapsing is one of the most common emotional obstacles encountered in recovery. Anxiety may arise from the thought of reverting to previous behaviors or encountering obstacles in their advancement. This worry can be crippling, affecting one's mental health and possibly impeding the healing process. Establishing a resilient attitude and fostering emotional stability requires acknowledging and resolving this fear.

ADAPTIVE TECHNIQUES

Managing emotional difficulties during rehabilitation requires the development of strong coping mechanisms. Cultivating self-awareness and mindfulness is one strategy. People can learn to better understand their emotions and respond to them in more productive ways by engaging in mindfulness practices. By practicing mindfulness, people might lessen the emotional toll that regrets from the past or anxieties about the future take on them.

Creating wholesome routines and habits is another essential coping mechanism. Stability can be greatly enhanced by creating a regular daily routine that includes activities that support mental, emotional, and physical health.

Essential elements that promote emotional resilience are enough sleep, a healthy diet, and regular exercise. Playing games that make you happy and fulfilled can also be a healthy way to let your emotions out.

In addition, adopting a self-compassionate perspective is essential for managing emotional difficulties. People must be compassionate and patient toward themselves on their journey toward recovery, which may include setbacks. Relying on life lessons instead of obsessing over past mistakes makes one's emotional state more resilient and upbeat.

LOOKING FOR ASSISTANCE

Maintaining emotional well-being requires understanding that healing is a team effort rather than a solo undertaking. Reaching out to friends, family, or support groups gives them access to a network of people who can relate to them and offer encouragement. Being honest about emotional difficulties creates a sense of community and lessens the weight of going it alone.

Another important component of emotional health throughout rehabilitation is professional support. Professionals with training in addiction or mental health, such as therapists or counselors, can provide customized advice and therapeutic approaches. These specialists offer a secure environment where people may investigate and deal with the underlying emotional problems that are causing their difficulties, which promotes a more thorough healing process.

Emotional well-being during the recovery process is influenced by several interconnected factors, including identifying emotional difficulties, putting good coping mechanisms into practice, and actively seeking help. Since every person's journey is different, by accepting these ideas, people can build a resilient foundation for long-lasting recovery and traverse their emotional landscape with resilience.

CHAPTER NINE

EXTENDED-TERM NUTRITIONAL ASPECTS

NUTRITION FOLLOWING RECUPERATION

After Healing Long-term health depends critically on nutrition, particularly for those who have experienced disease, surgery, or other medical procedures. The body may require more nutrition during the healing phase, therefore eating should be done with purpose. It's common knowledge that eating enough protein will aid in muscle growth and tissue healing. Vital nutrients, such as vitamins and minerals, are crucial for the body's healing processes because they support general health and immune system strength.

When it comes to post-recovery nutrition, water is just as important as protein and other necessary elements. Maintaining proper hydration facilitates several physiological processes and helps the body flush out waste. After medical procedures, maintaining proper fluid balance is especially important because it can speed up the healing process.

SUSTAINING A HEALTHFUL WAY OF LIFE

A healthy lifestyle is something you have to commit to long after you've recovered. The cornerstone of a healthy lifestyle is consuming a diet rich in fruits, vegetables, whole grains, lean proteins, and balance. Another essential element is regular physical activity, which has many advantages including better weight management, elevated mood, and cardiovascular health. Incorporating stress-reduction strategies, getting enough sleep, and abstaining from bad habits like smoking also improve general well-being.

Maintaining a healthy lifestyle in the context of long-term dietary issues entails creating enduring habits. This involves controlling portion sizes, eating with awareness, and making thoughtful food selections. Incorporating a wide variety of nutrient-dense foods guarantees that the body gets a wide range of vital vitamins and minerals.

The development of these behaviors promotes longevity and resilience against future health issues.

OBSERVATION OF HEALTHCARE PROVIDERS

People managing long-term nutritional concerns, particularly those who have had medical procedures, must follow up with healthcare providers. Regular visits to medical specialists enable the tracking of general health and nutritional state. During these visits, it is possible to address any new issues that may arise, modify diet plans as needed, and make sure the person is headed in the right direction for long-term health.

Medical professionals can provide individualized guidance based on a patient's medical history, present ailments, and unique dietary requirements. They are essential in customizing dietary advice, offering advice on supplements when needed, and answering any queries or difficulties that may come up in the long-term and post-recovery stages.

www.ingramcontent.com/pod-product-compliance
Lightning Source LLC
Chambersburg PA
CBHW060815260726
48660CB00002B/955